Take A Bite

Endorsed, healthy, and complete Midweek Recipes

by

Lorna Fiorentini

Table of contents

5. Chickenpox Salad
6. Summer couscous salad

Chapter 3

Easiest Italian food

1. Italian seafood rice
2. Spanish tomato bread with jamón Serra
3. The best carbonara recipe for spaghetti
4. Baked Italian broccoli and salmon
5. Italian Meatloaf

Chapter 4

Delicious and Tasty cake recipe

1. Easy chocolate fudge cake
2. Carrot cake
3. Lemon drizzle cake
4. The finest chocolate cake

Introduction

Food gives me a lot of joy, curiosity, and comfort in my life. I've been in the culinary industry for 25 years and even owned my restaurant. I merged my passion for food and culinary talents with nutrition science to become a registered dietitian nutritionist, often known as an RDN. Currently, I teach graduate-level culinary nutrition classes in which my students and I create foods from across the world and analyze how culture, tradition, and local ingredients contribute to the creation of distinct cuisines. Along with my experience, I contribute my wealth of culinary knowledge, cooking abilities, and food enthusiasts to the recipes and advice in this book.

This cookbook was designed to be a useful tool in both your kitchen and the store.

Chapter 1

Incredible Soup For The Soul
Spiced carrot and lentil soup

A flavorful, spicy mixture that is also low in fat and rich in iron. It can be cooked in a slow cooker or in less than 30 minutes.

Ingredients

- 2 teaspoons cumin seeds one pinch red pepper flakes
- 2/TBS of olive oil
- 600 grams of cleaned and coarsely shredded carrots (no need to peel)
- 140 grams of red lentils divided

- Hot vegetable stock, 1 liter (from a cube is fine)
- 125ml milk (for dairy-free options, see "try" below)
- To be served: naan bread and plain yogur

Method

STEP 1

Two tablespoons of cumin seeds and a sprinkling of red chili flakes should be dry-fried for one minute or until they begin to leap around the pan and exude their scents.

STEP 2

Use a spoon to scoop out roughly half and set it aside. 600 grams of coarsely grated carrots, 140 grams of split red lentils, 1 liter of boiling vegetable stock, and 125 milliliters of milk should all be added to the pan and brought to a boil.

STEP 3

To soften and swell the lentils, simmer for 15 minutes.

STEP 4

Use a stick blender or a food processor to puree the soup (or leave it chunky if you prefer).

STEP 5

Add salt and pepper to taste. Add a dollop of plain yogurt and a sprinkle of the saved toasted spices to finish. With hot naan flatbread, serve.

Lentil soup

Enjoy this hearty red lentil, carrot, and leek soup that is vegetarian. It provides three of your daily five servings while being low in calories and fat.

Ingredients

- 2 liters of ham stock or veggie stock
- Red lentils, 150 g
- 6 carrots, cut finely
- Two medium leeks, thinly sliced (approximately 300g), plus a tiny amount of parsley, to serve

Method

STEP 1

Lentils are added to a big pan of simmering stock. Bring to a boil and give the lentils a few minutes to soften.

STEP 2

Add the carrots and leeks and season. If using ham stock, omit the salt since it will make the dish excessively salty. Once it comes to a boil, turns down the heat, covers the pot, and simmer for 45–1 hour, or until the lentils are tender. If desired, top with parsley and serve with buttered toast.

Italian vegetable soup

With this nutritious vegetable soup that is simple to freeze in advance, warm up your week.

Ingredients

- 2 chopped onions and 2 chopped carrots each
- 4 celery sticks, chopped
- 1 tablespoon of olive oil
- 2 tablespoons sugar
- 4 smashed garlic cloves
- 2 tablespoons of tomato purée
- 2 bay leaves and a few thyme sprigs
- 3 chopped courgettes, 400g of butter beans, and 400g of chopped tomatoes, all drained
- 1.2 liters of vegetable stock

- 100g of grated Parmesan or a vegetarian substitute
- 140 g of miniature pasta
- a tiny bunch of shredded basil

Method

STEP 1

In a large saucepan, gently sauté the onion, carrots, and celery in the oil for 20 minutes, or until tender. If they stick, splash water on them. When the courgettes begin to brown a little, add the sugar, garlic, purée, and herbs, and simmer for a further 4-5 minutes on medium heat

STEP 2

Add the beans, tomatoes, and stock. After 20 minutes, simmer. If you're freezing, stop immediately (for up to three months). If not, stir half the Parmesan and simmer the pasta for 6 to 8 minutes, or until it is done. To serve, top with remaining Parmesan and basil. If frozen, thaw and reheat first, then add the pasta and cheese and proceed as directed above.

Classic minestrone soup

Prepare this old vegetable soup made in the style of Italy, using noodles and a substantial tomato base. It is high in fiber and vitamin C and contains few calories.

Ingredients

- 3 tablespoons of extra virgin olive oil.
- 1 finely chopped onion
- 1 celery stick, cut finely

- 1 peeled and coarsely chopped carrot
- 1 chopped, coarsely diced courgette
- Smoked pancetta, 70g, diced
- 1 big clove of smashed garlic
- Dried oregano, 1/2 tsp.
- 1 cannellini bean, 400 g
- 400 g of chopped tomatoes in one can
- 2 tablespoons of tomato purée
- Vegetable stock, 1.2 liters
- 70g of tiny pasta and 1 bay leaf
- 100g greens, preferably kale, chard, or cavolo nero
- a serving of finely grated Parmesan and basil

Method

STEP 1

For 10 minutes, gently sauté the onion, celery, carrot, courgette, and pancetta in the oil in a large saucepan or casserole pot over low to medium heat. For one minute, add the oregano and garlic. Add the puréed tomatoes, stock, bay leaf, beans, and chopped tomatoes. According to taste. 30 minutes of simmering and cooking.

STEP 2

Cook the pasta and greens for an additional 10 minutes. Pour into bowls and top with some parmesan and basil.

Versatile veggies soup

Try a basic soup recipe that you can modify to include whatever vegetables you have on hand. Add creme fraiche and fresh herbs before serving.

Ingredients

- 700 ml stock, crème fraîche, and fresh herbs
- 300 g cubed potatoes

- 200 g chopped vegetables, including celery, onions, and carrots
- 1 tbsp oil.

Method

STEP 1

Heat the oil in a pan and fry the veggies and potatoes for a few minutes or until they start to soften.

STEP 2

Cover the vegetables with the stock and cook for 10 to 15 minutes or until they are soft. Season after blending until smooth. Serve with some fresh herbs and a dollop of crème fraîche. Will keep frozen for a month maximum.

RECIPES GUIDE

PUT SOUP IN A MAKER

Put all of your components in a soup maker to produce a great soup quickly while saving time and effort.

Chapter 2

Mouth Warming Delicacy

Tasty instant Pesto 10 minutes couscous salad

This is deliciously served straight from the refrigerator at home and makes a nice lunchbox filling for outings.

Ingredients

- 200ml of boiling, low-salt vegetable stock and 100g of couscous (from a cube is fine)
- two onions, spring
- 1 pepper, red
- 1 cucumber
- 50g of cubed feta cheese
- 2 tablespoons of Pesto
- 2 tablespoons pine nuts

Method

STEP 1

Place the stock on top of the couscous in a big bowl. Cover and cook for 10 minutes, until fluffy and the stock has completely absorbed. Slice the pepper and onions, then dice the cucumber, all while you wait. Add these to the couscous, stir the Pesto and feta with a fork, and then top with pine nuts to serve.

Chicken satay salad

Try this flavorful, low-effort midweek dinner for high protein content. Chicken breasts should be marinated before being drizzled with a flavorful peanut sauce.

Ingredients

- 1 tablespoon of tamari
- Medium curry powder, 1 teaspoon
- ¼ teaspoon ground cumin and 1 grated garlic clove
- 1 teaspoon pure honey
- 2 chicken breast fillets without skin (or use turkey breast)
- a tablespoon of crunchy peanut butter (choose a sugar-free version with no palm oil, if possible)
- 1 tablespoon of sweet chili sauce

- 10 ml of lime juice
- Sunflower oil is used to clean the pan.
- 2 wedges of Little Gem lettuce hearts
- Sliced and halved 1/4 cucumber
- 1 banana, 1 shallot, 1/2 pomegranate, 12 coriander, and thinly sliced

Method

STEP 1

Put the curry powder, cumin, garlic, and honey into a big bowl with the tamari. Mix well. Cut the chicken breasts in half horizontally to create a total of four fillets. Add the chicken to the marinade and thoroughly combine to coat. To allow the flavors to permeate the chicken, leave it in the refrigerator for at least one hour or overnight.

STEP 2

Create a spoonable sauce by combining the peanut butter, lime juice, and chili sauce in the meantime. Add a little oil to a sizable nonstick frying pan when cooking the chicken. Add the chicken, cover with a lid, and cook over medium heat for 5–6 minutes, turning the fillets over for the final minute until done but moist. For a little period of rest, place aside covered.

STEP 3

Toss the lettuce wedges with the cucumber, shallot, coriander, and pomegranate while the chicken rests. Pile the salad into plates. Add a little sauce on top. Spread the remaining sauce on top of the salad after slicing the chicken. Consume the chicken while it is still warm.

Greek salad

Quickly prepare a vibrant, fresh Greek salad. It goes well with grilled meats at a barbeque or by itself as a main course vegetable.

Ingredients

- large vine tomatoes, sliced into irregular wedges
- 1 cucumber, peeled and deseeded, then roughly chopped 12 thinly sliced red onion
- 16 olives, Kalamata
- 1 teaspoon dried oregano
- 85g feta cheese, chunked (barrel matured feta is the best)
- 4 tbsp extra virgin Greek olive oil

Method

STEP 1

In a large mixing bowl, combine 4 large vine tomatoes, cut into wedges, 1 peeled, deseeded, and chopped cucumber, 12 thinly sliced red onions, 16 Kalamata olives, 1 teaspoon dried oregano, 85g feta cheese chunks, and 4 tablespoons Greek extra virgin olive oil.

STEP 2
Season lightly, then serve with crusty bread to soak up the juices.

Next level potato salad
With our ultimate version of this ever-versatile side dish, you can take the humble potato salad to the next level. It's ideal for picnics, barbecues, and other outdoor activities.

Ingredients

- 800g Jersey Royals, Charlotte or Anya potatoes, or another waxy potato variety
- 2 tablespoons wholegrain mustard
- 2 tablespoons muscatel vinegar or white wine vinegar
- 4 tablespoons olive oil
- 1 very finely chopped shallot
- 3 tablespoons mayonnaise
- 2 tablespoons soured cream
- 1 tablespoon of horseradish sauce
- ¼ lemon juice
- 2 spring onions, finely sliced

Method

STEP 1

is to place the potatoes in a sizable pan of salted, ice-cold water. Bring to a boil, then simmer for 10 minutes or until the vegetables are fork-tender.

STEP 2

Stir the mustard, vinegar, olive oil, and shallot with a generous amount of salt and freshly ground pepper while the potatoes are cooking. When the potatoes are cool enough to handle, peel them if you'd like, chop them in half, quarters, or, if they're large, into bite-sized pieces before tossing them in the mustard dressing and coating them completely. Allow to totally cool.

STEP 3

In the meantime, combine the mayonnaise, soured cream, horseradish, and lemon juice. When the potatoes have cooled, combine them with the spring onions in the mayonnaise mixture. Just before serving, spoon into a dish and top with the crispy onions, or provide the crispy onions on the side for guests to sprinkle over their plates.

Chickpea Salad

A nutritious chickpea salad can be spiced up with a dash of harissa. It can be prepared in about ten minutes and is the perfect complement to slow-cooked Greek lamb.

Ingredients

- 400g canned chickpeas, drained and rinsed 1 red onion, thinly sliced 2 large tomatoes, diced
- 2 tablespoons olive oil
- 2 tablespoons harissa
- 1 lemon, freshly squeezed

Method

STEP 1

Combine all the ingredients, crushing a little so the chickpeas are a little rough around the edges - this helps absorb the dressing. (Can be made a day ahead and refrigerated.)

Summer couscous salad

This simple, hearty couscous salad captures the flavors of summer. It's ideal for an al fresco brunch with fried halloumi, vine tomatoes, and courgettes.

Ingredients

- 250g couscous, 250ml vegetable stock, boiled 400g can chickpeas, drained and rinsed
- 1 to 2 tablespoons vegetable or olive oil
- 300g courgette, slanted sliced
- 250g bag halloumi cheese, thickly sliced and then divided lengthways 300g tiny vine-ripened tomatoes halve.

To make the dressing
- 1 litre olive oil

- 3 tablespoons lime juice
- 2 finely minced big garlic cloves
- 2 tbsp fresh mint, chopped

- ½ teaspoon sugar

Method

STEP 1

Place the couscous in a bowl, pour in the boiling stock, and mix thoroughly with a fork. Leave for 4 minutes, covered with a plate. Meanwhile, combine all of the dressing ingredients in a mixing dish. Fluff the couscous with a fork, then stir in the chickpeas and half of the dressing. Mix and spoon into a wide serving plate.

STEP 2

Heat 1 tablespoon oil in a big frying pan over high heat, then cook the courgette slices for 2 to 3 minutes, or until they are dark golden brown. Onto kitchen paper, lift out. Put the tomatoes in the pan cut-side down and cook for a further couple of minutes, or until the undersides start to turn golden. The tomatoes are placed on top of the couscous before the courgettes.

STEP 3

If the pan is dry, add some more oil and heat it. Add the halloumi strips and cook for 2-3 minutes, flipping them occasionally until they are crisp and sizzling brown. Sprinkle the remaining dressing over the tomatoes before stacking them on top. As soon as you can, serve.

Chapter 3

Easiest Italian food Recipes
Italian seafood rice

Because the mixed seafood is already prepared, assembling this dish couldn't be simpler.

Ingredients

- Olive oil
- one tablespoon
- Sliced 110g of chorizo meat and 1 leek or onion
- ½ tsp of turmeric
- Long grain rice, 300g
- 1l hot chicken or fish stock
- Frozen peas, 200g

- 400g of defrosted frozen seafood mixture

Method
STEP 1

Leeks should be softened for five minutes without browning in hot oil in a deep frying pan. Chorizo should be added and fried until it releases its oils. After coating the rice and turmeric with the oils, add the stock. Stirring occasionally, bring to a boil, then simmer for 15 minutes.

STEP 2

Add the peas and cook for 5 minutes. Stir in the seafood and cook for 1 to 2 minutes, or until the rice is tender. After seasoning, serve the dish right away with lemon wedges.

RECIPES GUIDE
SAUAGE CHORIZO

Spanish chorizo sausage has a smoked paprika flavor and is from that country. Instead, use a few pieces of pig or chicken, cooking them for 5 minutes with 1 teaspoon of smoky paprika before adding the rice.

Spanish tomato bread with jamón Serrano

These delectable tapas nibbles can be prepared in just five minutes and are the ideal addition to a drinks party.

Ingredients

- 4 chopped ripe tomatoes
- 1 chopped clove of garlic
- 3 tbsp olive oil, salt, and pepper
- 20 baguette slices
- 5 to 6 slices of Serrano Ham

Methods

STEP 1

Combine the chopped tomatoes with the garlic clove, extra virgin olive oil, salt, and pepper. Until needed, keep in the refrigerator.

STEP 2

Toast 20 baguette slices before serving. Each piece of bread should have a small amount of tomato topping. One piece of jamón Serrano should be placed on each slice of bread after chopping up 5–6 slices of the ham.

RECIPES AND SHOPPING ADVICE

Prosciutto is similar to jamón serrano, a Spanish ham that you might substitute even if it is slightly more expensive.

The best carbonara recipe for

spaghetti

Learn how to make delicious spaghetti carbonara. Italians love this cheesy pasta dish, and with the appropriate technique, you can prepare it flawlessly every time.

Ingredients

- 100 grams pancetta
- 3 big eggs 50g pecorino cheese 50g parmesan
- 350 grams pasta
- 2 plump garlic cloves, peeled and unpeeled
- 50g unsalted butter, sea salt, and black pepper, freshly ground

Methods

STEP 1

Bring a large saucepan of water to a

boil.

STEP 2

Finely cut the 100g pancetta, removing any rind first. Finely grate 50g pecorino cheese and 50g parmesan and combine.

STEP 3

In a medium mixing bowl, whisk together three big eggs and season with freshly grated black pepper. Set aside everything.

STEP 4

Add 1 teaspoon salt to the boiling water, then add 350g spaghetti and cook at a steady simmer, covered, for 10 minutes, or until al dente (just cooked).

STEP 5

Squash 2 peeled plump garlic cloves

with a knife blade to bruise them.

STEP 6

Fry the pancetta with the garlic while the pasta cooks. Place 50g unsalted butter in a large frying pan or wok and, once melted, add the pancetta and garlic.

STEP 7

Cook for about 5 minutes, stirring frequently, until the pancetta is brown and crisp. Because the garlic has now imparted its flavor, remove it with a slotted spoon and discard.

STEP 8

Keep the pancetta on a low heat. Lift the pasta from the water with a pasta fork or tongs and place it in the frying pan with the pancetta. Don't worry if some water drips into the pan (you want this to happen), and don't throw away the pasta water just yet.

STEP 9

Combine the majority of the cheese with the eggs, reserving a tiny quantity for subsequent sprinkling.

STEP 10

Remove the pan with the spaghetti and pancetta from the heat. Pour in the eggs and cheese rapidly. Lift up the spaghetti with tongs or a long fork so it readily mixes with the egg mixture, which thickens but does not scramble, and everything is coated.

STEP 11

To keep it saucy, add more pasta cooking water (several tablespoons should do it).

You only want it moist, not wet. If necessary, season with salt.

STEP 12

Twist the spaghetti onto the serving dish or bowl with a long-pronged fork. Serve immediately with a dusting of the remaining cheese and black pepper to taste. If the dish becomes too dry before serving, add little additional hot pasta water to recover the glossy sauciness.

RECIPE SUGGESTIONS
THE MYSTERY INGREDIENT...

As you move the spaghetti to the heated frying pan, dribble in some pasta water. Everything comes together to form a light, silky smooth sauce.

Baked Italian broccoli and salmon

This velvety pasta bake gives broccoli a new lease on life.

Ingredients

- 250g penne 300g broccoli (cut into big florets)
- 25g butter 25g all-purpose flour
- 600ml of milk
- Mascarpone 100g
- 8 drained and thickly sliced sundried tomatoes (preserved in olive oil)
- 2 tablespoons tiny capers (optional) washed to get rid of extra salt or vinegar
- 8 anchovy fillets, cut in half (optional)
- 10 big freshly torn basil leaves
- 4 skinless fresh salmon fillets
- 50g finely grated mature cheddar

Methods

STEP 1

Preheat the oven to 190 degrees

Celsius/gas 5/fan 170 degrees Celsius and prepare an ovenproof dish (measuring 20 by 30cm and about 5cm deep). In the meantime, bring a big pot of water to a boil for the pasta. When the water is rapidly boiling, add the pasta and season generously with salt. Return to the boil and simmer for 6 minutes, stirring occasionally. Return the water to a boil, add the broccoli and cook for 4 minutes more, or until the broccoli is firm yet tender. Drain thoroughly.

STEP 2
While the pasta is cooking, combine the butter, flour, and milk in a large saucepan and heat, whisking or constantly stirring, until the sauce thickens and becomes smooth. Remove from the fire and whisk in the mascarpone, sun-dried tomatoes, capers

(if using), anchovies (if using), and basil, then season with salt and pepper.

STEP 3
Cut the salmon fillets in half widthwise (you'll notice an evident divide on each fillet), then arrange the pieces in a single layer on the base of the ovenproof dish. Top with the broccoli mixture and sprinkle with the shredded cheddar. (If you want to get ahead, chill this for up to 4 hours.)

STEP 4
Bake for 30 minutes, or until the mixture is pale golden and just starting to bubble around the edges - don't let it get too dark, or the fish will overcook.

Italian Meatloaf
This low-cost supper goes well with

jacket potatoes, green beans, and gravy.

Ingredients

- 50g freshly made white breadcrumbs
- 500g bag lean minced beef
- 4 tbsp coarsely grated Parmesan
- 1 finely chopped onion
- 100g pancetta
- cut 1 garlic clove minced
- 1 egg, beaten
- 1 tablespoon tomato purée

Methods

STEP 1
Preheat the oven to 190°C/170°C fan/gas 5. 5. Line the long sides and bottom of a 2-pound loaf pan with double-thick baking paper. In a separate bowl,

combine 2 tbsp breadcrumbs and Parmesan and set aside. Mix all of the remaining ingredients in a large mixing basin, seasoning with salt and pepper to taste.

STEP 2
Press the batter into the loaf pan and top with the remaining crumb mixture. 40-45 minutes, or until the top is brown and crispy. If the top does not brown in the oven, place the tin under the grill for 5 minutes. Allow cooling for 5 minutes in the tin before removing with the parchment and placing on a board. Serve with sliced potatoes and green beans.

Chapter 4

Delicious and Tasty cake recipes

Easy chocolate fudge cake
Need a crowd-pleasing cake that's also

simple to make? This super-squishy chocolate fudge cake with silky icing is a baking success.

Ingredients

- 150 ml sunflower oil plus additional for the tin
- Self-raising flour, 175g
- 2 tbsp cocoa powder
- Bicarbonate of soda, 1 teaspoon
- 150 g of caster sugar
- 2 tbsp. of golden syrup
- 2 big, lightly beaten eggs
- semi-skimmed milk, 150 ml.

To make the frosting

- Unsalted butter, 100g
- 225 grams of sugar
- 40g of cocoa butter

- Milk, 2 12 tbsp (a little more if needed)

Method

STEP 1

Oven temperature: 180°C/160°F fan/gas 4. Two 18cm sandwich tin bases should be lined and oiled. Sift the flour, cocoa powder, and baking soda in a bowl. Mix thoroughly after adding the caster sugar.

STEP 2

Create a well in the center and pour in the milk, eggs, sunflower oil, and golden syrup. Until smooth, beat vigorously with an electric whisk.

STEP 3

Fill the two tins with the mixture, and bake for 25–30 minutes, until the loaves are risen and are firm to the touch. Turn out onto a cooling rack after being taken out of the oven and chilling for 10 minutes.

STEP 4

Beat the unsalted butter in a bowl until it is soft to make the frosting. Add enough milk to make the icing frothy and spreadable, then gradually sieve and whisk in the icing sugar and cocoa powder.

STEP 5

Use the butter frosting to sandwich the two cakes together, and add extra icing to the top and sides of the cake.

Carrot cake

Enjoy an afternoon tea with friends that

includes this simple carrot cake. The cake can be baked, frozen, and then simply iced the following day.

Ingredients

- 175 grams of mild muscovado sugar
- 175ml sunflower seed oil
- 3 big, gently beaten eggs
- 140g carrot, grated (about 3 medium)
- 100 grams raisins
- 1 big orange, peeled and zested
- 175 grams of self-rising flour
- 1 tablespoon bicarbonate of soda
- 1 teaspoon cinnamon powder
- ½ teaspoon grated nutmeg (freshly grated will give you the best flavor)

For the icing

- 1½— 2 tbsp orange juice
- 175g icing sugar

Method

STEP 1
Preheat the oven to 180°C/160°C fan/gas mark 1. 4. Lightly grease and line an 18cm square cake pan with baking paper.

STEP 2
Mix the sugar, sunflower oil, and eggs in a large mixing bowl. Mix lightly with a wooden spoon. Combine the carrots, raisins, and orange zest in a mixing bowl.

STEP 3
Sift the flour, baking soda, cinnamon, and nutmeg into a mixing basin. Combine everything; the mixture will be soft and almost runny.

STEP 4

Pour the batter into the prepared pan and bake for 40-45 minutes, until the center feels firm and springy when pressed.

STEP 5

Allow cooling in the tin for 5 minutes before turning out, peeling off the paper, and cooling on a wire rack. (At this stage, you can freeze the cake if you want to serve it later.)

STEP 6

In a small bowl, whisk together the icing sugar and orange juice until smooth - the icing should be roughly the consistency of single cream. Place the cake on a serving platter and generously spread the frosting in diagonal lines across the top, allowing it to trickle down the edges.

Lemon drizzle cake

 It's impossible to finish this traditional lemon drizzle in one sitting, so why not make two?

Ingredients

- 225g softened unsalted butter
- 225 grams of sugar
- 225g of self-raising flour, 4 eggs
- zested lemon, one
- 85g of caster sugar and 112 lemons were juiced for the drizzle topping.
- 85g caster sugar and 112 lemons juiced for the drizzling topping

Method

STEP 1
Oven temperature set to 180°C/160°F fan/gas 4

STEP 2
When the butter and caster sugar is light and creamy, add the eggs one at a time, carefully incorporating each addition.

STEP 3
Sift in the self-rising flour and stir in the lemon zest after that.

STEP 4
Spoon the batter into a greaseproof paper–lined loaf pan (8 x 21 cm), leveling the top with a spoon, and bake.

STEP 5

Bake the cake for 45 to 50 minutes until an inserted thin skewer comes out clean.

STEP 6

Prepare the drizzle by combining the lemon juice and caster sugar while the cake cools in its pan.

STEP 7

7 Prick the heated cake with a fork or skewer, then sprinkle the glaze on top. The liquid will soak the cake, and the sugar will crisp up to make a wonderful topping.

STEP 8

Continue to cool completely in the tin before removing and serving.

The finest chocolate cake

Enjoy this deliciously moist, rich, and fudgy recipe for the best chocolate cake. Excellent for a party or afternoon tea.

Ingredients

- 200g dark chocolate (about 60% cocoa solids), 200g butter, cubed 1 tablespoon instant coffee granules
- 14 teaspoon bicarbonate of soda 85g self-raising flour 85g plain flour
- 200g muscovado light sugar
- 200g caster sugar, golden
- 25 grams of cocoa powder
- 3 large eggs
- 75 mL of buttermilk
- To decorate, use 50g grated chocolate or 100g curls

For Ganache

- 200g dark chocolate, around 60% cocoa solids, chopped, and 300ml double cream

- Golden caster sugar, 2 tablespoons

Methods

STEP 1

Preheat the oven to 160°C/140°F/gas. 3.
Butter and line a circular cake pan with
20 cm (7.5cm deep).

STEP 2

Add 200g of chopped dark chocolate and
200g of butter to a medium pan.

STEP 3

Pour 125ml of cold water and 1 tbsp of
instant coffee granules into the pan.

STEP 4

Gently warm everything over low heat, but don't let it get too hot. Alternately, microwave the mixture for about 5 minutes while stirring midway.

STEP 5

Combine and smooth out any lumps in the ingredients: 25g cocoa powder, 200g light muscovado sugar, 200g golden caster sugar, 85g self-raising flour, and 14 tsp bicarbonate of soda.

STEP 6

Combine 75ml of buttermilk with 3 medium eggs.

STEP 7

Combine the flour mixture, the egg mixture, and the melted chocolate mixture. Stir until the mixture is smooth and fairly liquid.

STEP 8

Pour this mixture into the pan and bake for 1 hour 25 to 1 hour 30 minutes. Don't worry if it breaks a little bit. If you insert a skewer into the center, it should come out clean, and the top should feel solid.

STEP 9

Allow the cake cool in the tin (don't worry if it sinks a little), then remove it and let it cool entirely on a wire rack. Slice the chilled cake into three pieces horizontally.

STEP 10

Place 200g of finely chopped dark chocolate in a bowl to start the ganache. Two tablespoons of golden caster sugar and 300ml of double cream should be added to a pan and heated until it is ready to boil.

STEP 11

Remove from the heat and pour over the chocolate. Stir the ingredients until the chocolate has melted and it is smooth. Cool until slightly thickened but still pourable.

STEP 12

Sandwich the layers together with a small amount of ganache. Pour the remainder over the cake, allowing it to drip down the edges and smoothing up any gaps with a palette knife.

STEP 13

Top with 50g grated chocolate or 100g chocolate curls to finish. The cake stays moist and sticky for 3-4 days

Conclusion

Check out some favorite Italian dishes to create for each occasion, such as holiday recipes, quick and simple dinners, healthy breakfast and lunch options, and more. Also included are the greatest culinary ideas.

9 798846 657151